Cobenfy: A Comprehensive Guide

Eugenia Barber

Copyright

All rights reserved.

No part of this publication may be reproduced, distributed, or transmitted in any form or by any means, including photocopying, recording, or other electronic or mechanical methods, without the prior written permission of the publisher, except in the case of brief quotations embodied in critical reviews and certain other noncommercial uses permitted by copyright law

© *2024 by Eugenia Barber*

Table of content

Introduction to Cobenfy

   What is Cobenfy?

   The Journey to FDA Approval

   The Need for a New Schizophrenia Treatment

Chapter 1

Understanding Schizophrenia

   Overview of Schizophrenia

   Challenges in Current Treatments

Chapter 2

The Science Behind Cobenfy

   Mechanism of Action: Xanomeline and Trospium Chloride

   How Cobenfy Targets M1 and M4 Receptors

   Differentiation from Atypical Antipsychotics

Chapter 3

Safety Information and Side Effects

   Common Adverse Reactions

   Contraindications and Warnings

   Monitoring and Management of Side Effects

Chapter 4

Dosage and Administration

    Available Dosage Forms and Strengths

    Recommended Dosing Guidelines

    Adjustments for Special Populations

Chapter 5

Patient Support and Accessibility

    Cobenfy Cares™ Program Overview

    Cost and Insurance Considerations

Chapter 6

Cobenfy in Context

    Comparison with Existing Treatments

    Addressing Unmet Needs in Schizophrenia Care

    Perspectives from Healthcare Providers

Chapter 7

Potential Risks and Limitations

    Risks in Special Populations (e.g., Renal/Hepatic Impairment)

    Anticholinergic CNS Effects

    Monitoring for Gastrointestinal and Cardiovascular Effects

Chapter 8

Future Directions in Neuropsychiatry

- Implications for Schizophrenia Treatment Paradigms
- Ongoing Research and Development
- Expanding Applications for Cobenfy

Frequently Asked Questions
- Common Concerns About Cobenfy
- Guidance for Patients and Caregivers
- Insights for Healthcare Professionals

Conclusion
- The Role of Cobenfy in Transforming Schizophrenia Care
- The Path Forward for Patients and Providers

Introduction to Cobenfy

What is Cobenfy?

Cobenfy (xanomeline and trospium chloride) is a groundbreaking medication designed to treat schizophrenia in adults. Developed by Bristol Myers Squibb, it represents the first new class of schizophrenia treatments in over three decades. Unlike traditional antipsychotic medications, Cobenfy introduces a novel pharmacological approach by selectively targeting M1 and M4 muscarinic acetylcholine receptors in the brain. These receptors are implicated in modulating cognitive and psychotic symptoms, making them a key focus for advancing schizophrenia care.

Cobenfy is a combination of two components:

- Xanomeline, a muscarinic receptor agonist that primarily acts on M1 and M4 receptors in the central nervous system.
- Trospium chloride, a muscarinic receptor antagonist that prevents peripheral side effects by acting outside the brain.

By avoiding the dopamine D2 receptor pathways targeted by most antipsychotics, Cobenfy reduces the likelihood of many common side effects associated with schizophrenia treatments, such as movement disorders and metabolic complications. This unique mechanism not only improves symptom management but also broadens the scope of treatment options for patients who have struggled with inadequate responses or intolerable side effects from existing therapies.

The Journey to FDA Approval

The development of Cobenfy is a story of persistence and innovation. After years of limited advancements in schizophrenia pharmacology, Bristol Myers Squibb conducted a comprehensive research program to explore muscarinic receptor modulation. The culmination of this effort was the EMERGENT clinical trial program, which provided the foundation for Cobenfy's approval.

The EMERGENT trials included three placebo-controlled efficacy studies and two long-term open-label studies. In the pivotal Phase 3 trials, EMERGENT-2 and EMERGENT-3, Cobenfy demonstrated statistically significant improvements in schizophrenia symptoms compared to placebo, as measured by the Positive and Negative Syndrome Scale (PANSS). These studies also established the drug's safety and tolerability, with common adverse effects like nausea, dyspepsia, and constipation being generally manageable.

The U.S. Food and Drug Administration (FDA) granted approval for Cobenfy in September 2024. This milestone was celebrated as a major advancement in neuropsychiatry, marking the reentry of Bristol Myers Squibb into this therapeutic area with a transformative treatment option. The approval also underscored the importance of innovation in addressing the diverse needs of schizophrenia patients.

The Need for a New Schizophrenia Treatment

Schizophrenia affects approximately 2.8 million people in the United States and nearly 24 million globally. It is a persistent and often disabling mental illness characterized by positive symptoms (e.g., hallucinations, delusions), negative symptoms (e.g., social withdrawal, lack of motivation), and cognitive impairments (e.g., memory deficits, poor concentration). Despite the availability of antipsychotic medications, up to 60% of patients experience inadequate symptom control or intolerable side effects.

Current treatments primarily focus on dopamine D2 receptor antagonism, a mechanism that has remained largely unchanged for decades. While effective for many, this approach often leads to significant side effects, including movement disorders, metabolic issues, and sedation, which can hinder adherence and quality of life. Furthermore, the heterogeneity of schizophrenia symptoms means that no single treatment works for all patients, creating a need for more targeted and flexible options.

Cobenfy's novel mechanism represents a paradigm shift in schizophrenia care. By leveraging muscarinic receptor modulation, it provides a fresh approach to symptom management that minimizes reliance on traditional pathways. This innovation addresses a critical unmet need in psychiatry, offering new hope to patients, caregivers, and healthcare providers seeking more effective and tolerable treatment options.

Chapter 1

Understanding Schizophrenia

Overview of Schizophrenia

Schizophrenia is a complex and persistent mental illness that affects how a person thinks, feels, and behaves. It is characterized by a range of symptoms that disrupt daily functioning, making it difficult for individuals to engage in meaningful activities, maintain relationships, and live independently. Schizophrenia typically manifests in early adulthood and affects approximately 2.8 million people in the United States and nearly 24 million globally. It is one of the top 15 leading causes of disability worldwide, reflecting its profound impact on individuals, families, and healthcare systems.

The exact cause of schizophrenia remains unknown, but research suggests a combination of genetic, neurobiological, and environmental factors. Changes in brain structure and chemistry, particularly involving dopamine and glutamate, are believed to play a role. Stress, trauma, and prenatal exposure to infections or malnutrition are also considered risk factors.

Diagnosing schizophrenia is challenging because its symptoms can overlap with other mental health conditions. Diagnosis typically requires the presence of symptoms for at least six months and significant impairment in social or occupational functioning. While there is no cure for schizophrenia, treatment can help manage symptoms and improve quality of life.

Symptom Domains: Positive, Negative, and Cognitive Symptoms

Schizophrenia symptoms are often categorized into three domains: positive, negative, and cognitive symptoms. Each domain affects individuals differently and contributes to the overall complexity of the disorder.

Positive Symptoms:

Positive symptoms are additions to normal mental functioning and include hallucinations, delusions, disorganized thinking, and disordered speech.

- Hallucinations: Sensory experiences that occur without external stimuli, such as hearing voices or seeing things that are not present.
- Delusions: Strongly held false beliefs, often involving paranoia or grandiosity.
- Disorganized Thinking: Difficulty organizing thoughts coherently, which may lead to tangential or nonsensical speech.

Negative Symptoms:

Negative symptoms involve a reduction or absence of normal behaviors and emotional expressions. These symptoms often have a profound impact on social functioning and quality of life.

- Affective Flattening: Reduced emotional expression or a flat affect.
- Anhedonia: Inability to experience pleasure from activities once enjoyed.
- Avolition: Lack of motivation to initiate or sustain purposeful activities.

- Social Withdrawal: Avoidance of social interactions and difficulty maintaining relationships.

Cognitive Symptoms:

Cognitive dysfunction is a core feature of schizophrenia that affects memory, attention, and decision-making.

- Impaired Attention: Difficulty focusing on tasks or maintaining concentration.
- Memory Deficits: Challenges in retaining and recalling information.
- Executive Dysfunction: Problems with planning, organizing, and problem-solving.

Cognitive symptoms are often the most disabling aspect of schizophrenia, significantly limiting a person's ability to work or function independently.

Challenges in Current Treatments

Despite advancements in pharmacology, managing schizophrenia remains a significant challenge. The primary treatment options are antipsychotic medications, which primarily target dopamine D2 receptors to reduce positive symptoms. While effective for many, these medications are not without limitations:

Side Effects:

- Many antipsychotics cause severe side effects, including weight gain, diabetes, sedation, and movement disorders (e.g., tardive dyskinesia). These side effects often lead to poor medication adherence.

Limited Efficacy for Negative and Cognitive Symptoms:

- Current treatments are less effective in addressing negative and cognitive symptoms, leaving many patients with significant functional impairments.

High Rates of Relapse:

- Up to 60% of patients experience inadequate symptom improvement or relapse due to discontinuation or switching therapies.

Individual Variability:

- Schizophrenia is a heterogeneous condition, meaning no single treatment works for everyone. This variability necessitates the development of novel therapies tailored to individual needs.

The emergence of treatments like Cobenfy, which target new pathways in the brain, holds promise for addressing these challenges and improving outcomes for individuals living with schizophrenia.

Chapter 2

The Science Behind Cobenfy

Mechanism of Action: Xanomeline and Trospium Chloride

Cobenfy (xanomeline and trospium chloride) is a novel medication developed for the treatment of schizophrenia. It combines two distinct pharmacological agents: xanomeline, a muscarinic receptor agonist, and trospium chloride, an antimuscarinic agent. This combination works in a unique way to target the underlying pathophysiology of schizophrenia.

Xanomeline:

Xanomeline is the key active ingredient in Cobenfy. It is a selective agonist for the muscarinic acetylcholine receptors, specifically M1 and M4. These receptors are part of the cholinergic system, which plays a crucial role in cognitive functions such as attention, memory, and executive function. By targeting these receptors, xanomeline aims to enhance cognitive function and alleviate certain symptoms of schizophrenia, particularly those related to negative and cognitive domains of the illness. Xanomeline's activity at M1 and M4 receptors is thought to improve neurotransmitter signaling, contributing to improved cognition and emotional regulation in patients with schizophrenia.

Trospium Chloride:

Trospium chloride is an antimuscarinic agent included in Cobenfy to help modulate the effects of xanomeline. However, unlike xanomeline, trospium chloride is a muscarinic receptor antagonist that primarily acts peripherally rather than in the brain. This component helps to mitigate any potential side effects that could arise from xanomeline's activity on muscarinic receptors outside of the central nervous system (CNS). Trospium chloride does not cross the blood-brain barrier effectively, which reduces the risk of central nervous system-related side effects that are commonly associated with muscarinic receptor antagonists.

Together, xanomeline and trospium chloride form a synergistic combination that targets schizophrenia's underlying neurochemical imbalances while minimizing side effects typically seen with other antipsychotic treatments.

How Cobenfy Targets M1 and M4 Receptors

Cobenfy distinguishes itself from traditional schizophrenia treatments by targeting the M1 and M4 muscarinic acetylcholine receptors. These receptors are part of the cholinergic system and play a vital role in cognitive and emotional processing.

M1 Receptors:

The M1 muscarinic receptor is located predominantly in the cortex and hippocampus, areas of the brain that are crucial for cognition and memory. Activation of the M1 receptor has been shown to enhance cognitive function, improve memory, and reduce symptoms associated with cognitive dysfunction in schizophrenia. Cognitive impairment is a hallmark of the disease and often the most debilitating. By stimulating M1 receptors, xanomeline in Cobenfy aims to address this gap in treatment by improving attention, memory, and executive function in patients with schizophrenia.

M4 Receptors:

The M4 muscarinic receptor is predominantly found in the striatum and other regions involved in motor and emotional regulation. M4 receptor activation has been linked to improvements in mood and reduction in psychotic symptoms such as delusions and hallucinations. In schizophrenia, dysregulated dopamine transmission often leads to positive symptoms (hallucinations, delusions). By targeting M4 receptors, xanomeline helps normalize dopamine activity in the brain, which can contribute to a reduction in positive symptoms of schizophrenia.

The selective targeting of these receptors by Cobenfy provides a unique pharmacological approach that is distinct from conventional treatments. This approach is thought to reduce cognitive and emotional symptoms of schizophrenia while improving overall functioning.

Differentiation from Atypical Antipsychotics

Atypical antipsychotics, the mainstay of current schizophrenia treatment, work primarily by blocking dopamine D2 receptors in the brain, which is effective in managing positive symptoms (hallucinations, delusions). However, these drugs often fail to adequately address the negative and cognitive symptoms of the disorder and come with a variety of side effects, such as weight gain, metabolic syndrome, and movement disorders (e.g., tardive dyskinesia).

Cobenfy differentiates itself from atypical antipsychotics in several key ways

Non-Dopamine Targeting:

While atypical antipsychotics primarily block dopamine receptors to manage symptoms, Cobenfy works by targeting muscarinic receptors, specifically M1 and M4, without affecting dopamine receptors. This avoids many of the side effects associated with dopamine antagonism, such as movement disorders and sedation. Furthermore, by focusing on muscarinic receptors, Cobenfy addresses a different set of symptoms, particularly cognitive and negative symptoms, which are often inadequately treated by traditional antipsychotics.

Cognitive Benefits:

Atypical antipsychotics tend to have limited effects on cognitive symptoms. In contrast, Cobenfy's action at the M1 receptor is specifically aimed at enhancing cognition, making it potentially more effective for improving memory, attention, and executive function in people with schizophrenia.

Fewer Extrapyramidal Symptoms:

One of the challenges with atypical antipsychotics is the risk of extrapyramidal symptoms (EPS), which include movement disorders like tremors and rigidity. Cobenfy, by avoiding dopamine D2 receptor antagonism, may present a lower risk of these EPS, which are a significant concern for many patients on antipsychotic medications.

In summary, Cobenfy represents a groundbreaking approach to schizophrenia treatment, offering a new option for patients who may not respond well to traditional antipsychotics or who experience significant side effects. By targeting M1 and M4 receptors, it addresses cognitive and emotional symptoms with a novel mechanism that differs from conventional dopamine-based therapies.

Chapter 3

Safety Information and Side Effects

Common Adverse Reactions

Cobenfy (xanomeline and trospium chloride) is generally well-tolerated, but like all medications, it can cause adverse reactions. Some side effects are more common, and it's essential for healthcare providers and patients to be aware of them for appropriate management.

Gastrointestinal Effects:

The most frequently reported adverse reactions are related to the gastrointestinal (GI) system. Patients taking Cobenfy may experience nausea (19% vs. 4% with placebo), dyspepsia (18% vs. 5%), and constipation (17% vs. 7%). Vomiting (15% vs. 1%) is also common, though less frequent. These GI issues are consistent with the cholinergic effects of xanomeline and the antimuscarinic effects of trospium chloride, which can influence gut motility and digestion. Monitoring and supportive care may be necessary to manage these symptoms, especially in the initial phase of treatment.

Cardiovascular Effects:

Cobenfy can also lead to hypertension (11% vs. 2% with placebo) and tachycardia (5% vs. 2%). These cardiovascular side effects may require close monitoring of blood pressure and heart rate, particularly in patients with pre-existing cardiovascular conditions.

Abdominal Discomfort:

Abdominal pain (8% vs. 4%) is another commonly observed side effect. Patients may report discomfort or bloating, which could be a result of gastrointestinal irritation or motility changes.

Central Nervous System Effects:

As with many medications that influence the muscarinic system, CNS effects such as dizziness (5% vs. 2%) may occur. In some cases, these effects can lead to sedation or disorientation. Additionally, although rare, confusion or hallucinations can also occur, particularly in elderly patients or those with pre-existing neurological conditions.

Gastroesophageal Reflux Disease (GERD):

Gastroesophageal reflux disease (5% vs. <1%) has been reported in a small percentage of patients, likely due to the antimuscarinic properties of trospium chloride, which can relax the lower esophageal sphincter and promote acid reflux.

Contraindications and Warnings

Cobenfy is contraindicated in several conditions where its use may lead to serious or even life-threatening consequences. These include:

Urinary Retention:

Cobenfy can cause urinary retention, especially in older adults or those with a history of bladder outlet obstruction (e.g., benign prostatic hyperplasia). It is contraindicated in patients with pre-existing urinary retention and should be used with caution in those with clinically significant bladder issues.

Hepatic Impairment:

Cobenfy is not recommended for patients with moderate to severe liver impairment. Patients with Child-Pugh Class B or C liver dysfunction have higher systemic exposure to xanomeline, increasing the risk of adverse effects. It is important to assess liver function before initiating therapy and during treatment.

Narrow-Angle Glaucoma:

Cobenfy can cause pupillary dilation, which may trigger an acute angle-closure attack in patients with narrow-angle glaucoma. It is contraindicated in patients with untreated narrow-angle glaucoma.

Hypersensitivity Reactions:

Cobenfy is contraindicated in patients with a history of hypersensitivity to xanomeline or trospium chloride. Angioedema has been reported in some cases, and reactions can be severe, including swelling of the face, lips, tongue, or throat, which may interfere with breathing.

Gastric Retention:

Due to its antimuscarinic properties, Cobenfy can cause gastric retention, leading to the risk of gastrointestinal obstruction. It should not be used in patients with this condition.

Monitoring and Management of Side Effects

Given the potential for side effects with Cobenfy, healthcare providers should actively monitor patients during treatment and intervene when necessary. Proper management can help mitigate risks and improve the patient's quality of life.

Monitoring Gastrointestinal Effects:

Patients should be closely monitored for nausea, constipation, and other gastrointestinal disturbances. Adjusting the dose or managing symptoms with adjunctive medications (e.g., anti-nausea agents) may be necessary. In more severe cases, the dose may be reduced, or discontinuation may be considered if symptoms are unmanageable.

Cardiovascular Monitoring:

Routine monitoring of blood pressure and heart rate is crucial, especially for patients with existing hypertension or other cardiovascular issues. If significant increases in heart rate or blood pressure are observed, the healthcare provider may need to adjust the dose or evaluate for other underlying cardiovascular conditions.

Neurological Monitoring:

Central nervous system effects, such as dizziness or confusion, should be watched for, particularly in elderly patients or those with a history of neurological issues. Patients should be advised not to drive or operate heavy machinery until they know how Cobenfy affects them. If cognitive disturbances or hallucinations occur, a dose reduction or discontinuation of the drug may be warranted.

Urinary Retention and Renal Function:

As urinary retention is a significant risk, patients should be monitored for signs and symptoms, such as urinary hesitancy, weak stream, or incomplete bladder emptying. Reducing the dose or stopping the medication may be necessary if urinary retention occurs. Additionally, renal function should be evaluated, as patients with renal impairment are at higher risk for anticholinergic side effects.

Liver Function Monitoring:

Liver enzymes should be monitored before and during treatment, especially in patients with pre-existing liver conditions. Signs of liver dysfunction, such as jaundice or elevated liver enzymes, should prompt immediate discontinuation of the drug.

By following these safety protocols and maintaining close monitoring, healthcare providers can help ensure the safe and effective use of Cobenfy for patients with schizophrenia, minimizing risks while optimizing therapeutic outcomes.

Chapter 4

Dosage and Administration

Available Dosage Forms and Strengths

Cobenfy (xanomeline and trospium chloride) is available in capsule form and is prescribed for the treatment of schizophrenia in adults. The dosage forms and strengths provide flexibility in dosing to accommodate the needs of different patients based on their clinical response and tolerability.

Cobenfy is available in three strengths:

- 50 mg xanomeline / 20 mg trospium chloride
- 100 mg xanomeline / 20 mg trospium chloride
- 125 mg xanomeline / 30 mg trospium chloride

These varying strengths allow healthcare providers to tailor the medication to the individual patient's requirements, starting at a lower dose and titrating upward as needed. The formulation combines xanomeline, a muscarinic receptor agonist, with trospium chloride, an antimuscarinic agent that helps to balance the therapeutic effects while minimizing central nervous system side effects. The exact dosage may depend on factors such as the patient's severity of symptoms, comorbid conditions, and how well they tolerate the treatment.

Recommended Dosing Guidelines

Cobenfy is typically administered orally, with dosing recommendations designed to balance efficacy and safety for adults with schizophrenia. The recommended dosing guidelines are as follows:

Starting Dose:

- The initial recommended dose for most adults with schizophrenia is 50 mg xanomeline / 20 mg trospium chloride once daily. This allows the patient's body to adjust to the medication while minimizing the risk of common adverse effects such as gastrointestinal disturbances and dizziness.

Titration:

- The dosage can be gradually increased based on the patient's clinical response and tolerability. After the first week of therapy, the dose may be increased to 100 mg xanomeline / 20 mg trospium chloride once daily. Depending on the patient's tolerance and ongoing symptoms, the dose may be further increased to 125 mg xanomeline / 30 mg trospium chloride once daily. It is recommended that dosage adjustments be made no more frequently than every week.

Maximum Dose:

- The maximum recommended dose is 125 mg xanomeline / 30 mg trospium chloride once daily. This maximum dose is typically used for patients who have not experienced adequate symptom control with the lower doses or who can tolerate the higher dose without significant side effects.

Administration:

- Cobenfy should be taken with or without food. Capsules should be swallowed whole and not chewed, crushed, or opened to ensure the integrity of the formulation. Doses should be taken at the same time each day to help establish a routine and ensure consistent therapeutic levels in the bloodstream.

Adjustments for Special Populations

Certain populations may require dosage adjustments due to underlying health conditions, the potential for adverse effects, or altered drug metabolism. These populations include patients with hepatic or renal impairment, the elderly, and those with comorbid conditions.

Hepatic Impairment:

- Cobenfy should be used with caution in patients with mild hepatic impairment (Child-Pugh Class A). Although not specifically contraindicated, these patients may experience higher systemic exposure to xanomeline. Regular monitoring of liver enzymes is recommended to ensure safe use. For patients with moderate (Child-Pugh Class B) or severe (Child-Pugh Class C) hepatic impairment, Cobenfy is contraindicated due to the risk of increased adverse reactions.

Renal Impairment:

- Cobenfy is not recommended for patients with moderate or severe renal impairment (estimated glomerular filtration rate [eGFR] <60 mL/min). Trospium chloride, a component of Cobenfy, is primarily excreted by the kidneys. In patients with renal dysfunction, the drug's systemic exposure is significantly increased, which can elevate the risk of anticholinergic side effects like urinary retention, constipation, and dry mouth. For patients with mild renal impairment, the dose may be adjusted cautiously, with close monitoring of renal function and potential side effects.

Elderly Patients:

- Elderly patients are at a higher risk of experiencing anticholinergic effects such as dizziness, drowsiness, and urinary retention. Therefore, it is recommended that dosing be initiated at the lower end of the spectrum (50 mg xanomeline / 20 mg trospium chloride) to minimize risks. Close monitoring is essential, and the dosage may need to be adjusted more slowly based on the patient's response and tolerance.

Pregnancy and Lactation:

- Cobenfy has not been studied in pregnant or breastfeeding women, and its safety during pregnancy and lactation has not been established. The drug should be used during pregnancy only if the potential benefit justifies the potential risk to the fetus. Cobenfy is not recommended for use in breastfeeding women due to the unknown effects on the infant.

By following these dosing guidelines and making adjustments as necessary, healthcare providers can help ensure that Cobenfy is used safely and effectively for the treatment of schizophrenia in diverse patient populations. Regular monitoring is essential to detect and manage potential side effects, especially in patients with specific health conditions.

Chapter 5

Patient Support and Accessibility

Cobenfy Cares™ Program Overview

The Cobenfy Cares™ Program is a patient support initiative designed to assist individuals prescribed Cobenfy (xanomeline and trospium chloride) in managing their treatment journey. The program offers a range of services to help patients access, understand, and adhere to their prescribed medication. It aims to provide comprehensive support that addresses financial, logistical, and educational needs related to the medication.

Key features of the Cobenfy Cares™ Program include:

Personalized Support:

- The program assigns a dedicated Care Specialist to each participant, offering one-on-one support for navigating the process of obtaining Cobenfy. This includes explaining insurance coverage options, helping with any necessary paperwork, and answering questions about the medication's use and side effects.

Co-Pay Assistance:

- For patients with commercial insurance, Cobenfy Cares™ offers co-pay assistance to help reduce out-of-pocket expenses. Depending on the patient's insurance plan, the program may cover some or all of the co-pay, making the medication more affordable.

Patient Education:

- Through Cobenfy Cares™, patients receive educational materials that help them understand their condition, the role of Cobenfy in managing schizophrenia, and how to adhere to their treatment plan. This resource empowers patients to make informed decisions and actively engage in their treatment process.

Referrals and Support for Non-Commercial Insurance:

- In cases where a patient does not have commercial insurance, Cobenfy Cares™ may provide assistance through other channels, including patient assistance programs. These referrals help individuals find alternate routes to obtaining the medication, such as applying for financial aid through non-profit organizations or government programs.
- The Cobenfy Cares™ Program is designed to reduce the barriers to accessing care and provide patients with the resources needed for a successful treatment experience.

Cost and Insurance Considerations

The cost of Cobenfy can be a significant concern for patients, especially when they face high out-of-pocket expenses due to insurance deductibles, co-pays, or lack of insurance. Understanding the financial aspects of obtaining Cobenfy is crucial for ensuring access to treatment.

Insurance Coverage:

- Cobenfy is typically covered by major insurance plans, but the level of coverage can vary widely depending on the insurer and the patient's specific plan. Patients are encouraged to contact their insurance provider to confirm whether Cobenfy is included in their formulary and to verify any associated co-pays or coverage limitations. For many patients with commercial insurance, Cobenfy is covered under the specialty drug category, meaning it may require prior authorization or other steps to ensure coverage.

Co-Pay Assistance and Savings Programs:

- For patients who have insurance but still face high out-of-pocket costs, Cobenfy's Co-Pay Assistance Program through the Cobenfy Cares™ Program can help. The program typically provides financial assistance to patients who meet specific income and insurance criteria. This may include a reduction or complete coverage of the co-pay, making the medication more accessible for those who would otherwise struggle to afford it.

Cost Without Insurance:

- For uninsured patients, the cost of Cobenfy can be a significant barrier. The Patient Assistance Program (PAP) is designed to help such patients by offering the drug at reduced or no cost. Eligibility for the PAP is typically based on income and other factors, and patients are encouraged to apply for assistance as early as possible in their treatment journey.

Out-of-Pocket Considerations:

- It is important for patients to anticipate and plan for potential out-of-pocket costs associated with Cobenfy. Depending on the insurance plan and treatment plan, there may be additional charges such as clinic fees or drug administration costs. Patients are encouraged to discuss these costs upfront with their healthcare providers to understand their financial obligations and explore any available assistance options.

Accessing Assistance

- Getting access to Cobenfy is a critical part of the treatment process for patients with schizophrenia. While navigating insurance and financial concerns, the following steps can help ensure smooth access to the medication:

Navigating the Cobenfy Cares™ Program:

- To enroll in the Cobenfy Cares™ Program, patients can contact the program's support team through the program's website or by phone. Once enrolled, they can access the full range of services, including financial assistance, education, and personalized support.

Working with Healthcare Providers:

- Patients should work closely with their healthcare providers to ensure that their insurance covers Cobenfy or that they can obtain financial assistance through other means. Healthcare providers can also help facilitate the prior authorization process with insurance companies if necessary.

Patient Assistance Programs:

- For patients who do not have insurance or whose insurance does not cover Cobenfy, patient assistance programs like the Cobenfy Patient Assistance Program

(PAP) provide critical support. Patients can apply directly through the Cobenfy Cares™ Program to determine eligibility for free or discounted medication.

Online Resources and Support:

Patients can also access various online resources, including patient education materials, videos, and FAQs, to better understand their treatment options and how to navigate the system. Cobenfy Cares™ offers online tools and resources that patients and caregivers can use to stay informed and receive support.

By leveraging these support services, patients can improve their chances of successfully starting and continuing Cobenfy therapy, which can be crucial in managing schizophrenia effectively and improving their quality of life. The combination of financial assistance, educational resources, and personalized care makes it easier for patients to access and adhere to their prescribed treatment regimen.

Chapter 6

Cobenfy in Context

Comparison with Existing Treatments

Cobenfy (xanomeline and trospium chloride) represents a novel approach in the treatment of schizophrenia, a condition for which traditional antipsychotic treatments have dominated for decades. Most current treatments fall into two broad categories: typical antipsychotics and atypical antipsychotics. Typical antipsychotics, such as haloperidol, work primarily through dopamine receptor antagonism, while atypical antipsychotics like risperidone or olanzapine target a broader range of receptors, including serotonin and dopamine receptors.

While effective in managing certain aspects of schizophrenia, these drugs often come with significant limitations and side effects. Atypical antipsychotics, for example, are associated with metabolic side effects such as weight gain, diabetes, and lipid abnormalities, which can negatively impact patient adherence to treatment. Typical antipsychotics, although generally effective for positive symptoms like delusions and hallucinations, tend to have a higher incidence of extrapyramidal symptoms (EPS) and tardive dyskinesia (TD), both of which can be debilitating for patients.

In comparison, Cobenfy works through a different mechanism entirely, targeting the muscarinic acetylcholine receptors, specifically M1 and M4. By activating these receptors in the central nervous system, Cobenfy aims to address both positive and negative symptoms of schizophrenia without the extensive metabolic and motor side effects associated with traditional antipsychotics. This receptor-based mechanism provides a potentially more targeted approach, reducing the risk of side effects like weight gain, EPS, and TD, while providing therapeutic benefits for cognitive and emotional aspects of schizophrenia that are often neglected by existing treatments.

The combination of xanomeline and trospium chloride offers a unique advantage in balancing efficacy and safety. Xanomeline activates M1 and M4 receptors to enhance neurotransmission, while trospium chloride serves to limit peripheral effects, ensuring that the treatment acts predominantly within the central nervous system. This novel approach provides a promising alternative, particularly for patients who have struggled with the side effects of traditional antipsychotic medications.

Addressing Unmet Needs in Schizophrenia Care

Schizophrenia is a multifaceted condition that impacts various areas of a patient's life, including cognition, emotion, and social interactions. Despite advances in treatment over the years, there remain significant unmet needs in the care of individuals with schizophrenia. One of the most glaring gaps is the lack of treatments that address negative symptoms (such as social withdrawal, lack of motivation, and reduced emotional expression) and cognitive deficits (including memory issues, attention problems, and impaired decision-making). These aspects of the disease are not well-targeted by traditional antipsychotics, which tend to focus more on reducing positive symptoms like hallucinations and delusions.

Cobenfy's potential lies in its ability to target these previously neglected areas of schizophrenia. By stimulating M1 and M4 receptors in the brain, Cobenfy may help to improve cognition and emotional expression, providing a more holistic treatment option for schizophrenia. The drug's unique action also offers a way to potentially mitigate the cognitive dysfunction and negative symptoms that can severely impact a patient's quality of life and functional outcomes. This is a critical aspect in addressing the broader spectrum of symptoms and improving long-term prognosis for individuals with schizophrenia.

Another important aspect of schizophrenia treatment is improving patient adherence to medications. Many individuals with schizophrenia struggle with medication adherence due to side effects or concerns about long-term health implications. With Cobenfy's reduced risk of weight gain, metabolic issues, and motor symptoms, it may improve overall patient satisfaction and adherence, thus enhancing the likelihood of better treatment outcomes.

Perspectives from Healthcare Providers

Healthcare providers play a crucial role in the treatment of schizophrenia, and their perspectives on emerging therapies like Cobenfy are essential for understanding the broader impact of such treatments. In interviews and discussions with clinicians, many healthcare providers have expressed a growing need for treatments that go beyond simply controlling symptoms and work to improve the overall quality of life for patients.

For psychiatrists and clinicians treating schizophrenia, Cobenfy's efficacy in addressing both positive and negative symptoms is particularly promising. Many providers recognize that negative symptoms, such as social withdrawal and diminished emotional expression, are often underappreciated in treatment regimens. By offering a treatment that targets both these symptoms and cognitive impairments, Cobenfy aligns more closely with the multifaceted nature of schizophrenia, potentially allowing for better outcomes for patients.

Moreover, healthcare providers are encouraged by the safety profile of Cobenfy compared to traditional antipsychotics. With fewer metabolic side effects and a reduced risk of movement disorders like TD, Cobenfy offers an attractive alternative for patients who have struggled with the adverse effects of conventional medications. This is particularly relevant for elderly patients and individuals with comorbidities, who may face more pronounced side effects from other antipsychotic medications.

However, there is a degree of caution as well. While the early clinical trials have shown promise, healthcare providers continue to emphasize the need for long-term safety data to assess the full spectrum of Cobenfy's effects. In particular, the long-term effects on cognitive function, emotional regulation, and overall functional outcomes remain to be fully explored.

In conclusion, Cobenfy has the potential to change the landscape of schizophrenia treatment by offering a safer, more effective option that addresses the cognitive, negative, and positive symptoms of the disorder. As it gains wider acceptance in the healthcare community, it will be important to continue gathering real-world data and to ensure that providers are equipped with the necessary tools to integrate this novel treatment into their clinical practices.

Chapter 7

Potential Risks and Limitations

Risks in Special Populations (e.g., Renal/Hepatic Impairment)

Cobenfy (xanomeline and trospium chloride) offers significant promise for the treatment of schizophrenia, but like all medications, it carries risks, particularly in certain special populations. Patients with renal or hepatic impairment require particular attention when considering the use of Cobenfy due to the way its components are metabolized and eliminated from the body.

For renal impairment, trospium chloride, one of the key components of Cobenfy, is primarily excreted through the kidneys. As a result, individuals with moderate or severe renal impairment (those with an estimated glomerular filtration rate (eGFR) below 60 mL/min) may experience higher systemic exposure to the drug, which can lead to an increased incidence of adverse anticholinergic side effects such as dry mouth, constipation, urinary retention, and dizziness. As the body is less able to eliminate the drug effectively, these side effects could become more pronounced, potentially leading to discomfort or even more serious complications. Therefore, Cobenfy is not recommended in patients with moderate or severe renal impairment, and dose adjustments may be necessary for patients with milder renal impairment.

Similarly, for patients with hepatic impairment, the metabolism of xanomeline (the other active component of Cobenfy) may be altered, leading to higher systemic exposure to the drug. In patients with moderate or severe hepatic impairment, the use of Cobenfy could result in increased adverse reactions due to xanomeline's prolonged presence in the body. Therefore, Cobenfy is contraindicated in patients with moderate or severe hepatic impairment and is not recommended for those with mild hepatic impairment. Regular monitoring of liver function tests is necessary before and during treatment to identify potential issues early and to adjust dosing accordingly.

In both cases, healthcare providers must carefully assess renal and hepatic function before prescribing Cobenfy and may need to consider alternative treatments if these organs are significantly impaired.

Anticholinergic CNS Effects

One of the known risks associated with Cobenfy is the potential for central nervous system (CNS) anticholinergic effects due to the presence of trospium chloride, a muscarinic receptor antagonist. Trospium chloride's action on muscarinic receptors can lead to various CNS effects, including dizziness, confusion, hallucinations, and somnolence. These effects are particularly concerning in older patients, who may be more susceptible to the anticholinergic burden and its cognitive impact.

Patients with schizophrenia are already at heightened risk for cognitive deficits, and the additional cognitive side effects associated with Cobenfy may exacerbate this challenge. It is essential to monitor patients closely for signs of these CNS effects, especially during the initial stages of treatment or after dose increases. Providers should exercise caution when prescribing Cobenfy to individuals with a history of cognitive decline, delirium, or other CNS-related issues.

In addition, patients should be advised not to engage in activities that require mental alertness, such as driving or operating heavy machinery, until they are aware of how Cobenfy affects their cognition. If significant CNS side effects are observed, healthcare providers should consider adjusting the dose or discontinuing the medication to mitigate risks.

Monitoring for Gastrointestinal and Cardiovascular Effects

Gastrointestinal (GI) and cardiovascular effects are other important considerations in the safe use of Cobenfy. Cobenfy contains trospium chloride, which has known anticholinergic properties that can affect gastrointestinal motility. Patients may experience constipation, abdominal pain, nausea, or dyspepsia, which are relatively common adverse reactions associated with Cobenfy. Gastrointestinal motility can be significantly reduced in patients with gastrointestinal obstructive disorders, such as ulcerative colitis, intestinal atony, or myasthenia gravis. In these cases, Cobenfy should be used with caution, and healthcare providers may need to monitor for signs of gastric retention or other GI issues.

In some cases, if gastrointestinal symptoms become severe, it may be necessary to adjust the dosage or discontinue Cobenfy altogether. Providers should also consider the use of alternative treatments if GI side effects become problematic for patients.

Cobenfy can also have an impact on the cardiovascular system. One of the potential cardiovascular risks is an increase in heart rate, a side effect that has been observed during clinical trials. While generally mild, this increase in heart rate may not be appropriate for patients with certain cardiovascular conditions, such as hypertension or arrhythmias. It is important for healthcare providers to assess the patient's heart rate at baseline and regularly during treatment. If the heart rate becomes elevated or reaches unsafe levels, dose adjustments or discontinuation of the drug may be necessary.

The cardiovascular monitoring is especially important for patients with pre-existing heart conditions. Healthcare providers must weigh the risks and benefits of prescribing Cobenfy to these patients and should consider careful monitoring for any signs of adverse cardiovascular effects.

In conclusion, while Cobenfy offers significant promise as a treatment for schizophrenia, it is essential to recognize and manage the potential risks associated with its use, particularly in special populations, individuals at risk for anticholinergic CNS effects, and those vulnerable to gastrointestinal or cardiovascular complications. Careful screening, monitoring, and dose adjustments will help mitigate these risks and ensure the safety and efficacy of Cobenfy for each patient.

Chapter 8

Future Directions in Neuropsychiatry

Implications for Schizophrenia Treatment Paradigms

The introduction of Cobenfy (xanomeline and trospium chloride) to the schizophrenia treatment landscape marks an exciting potential shift in how the disorder is managed. Schizophrenia has long been treated with antipsychotic medications, primarily atypical antipsychotics, which address the positive symptoms of the disorder but often fall short when it comes to treating negative symptoms and cognitive impairments. Cobenfy's unique mechanism of action, targeting the M1 and M4 muscarinic receptors, offers a potential breakthrough in this regard.

By acting on muscarinic receptors in the brain, Cobenfy could address cognitive dysfunction, a central aspect of schizophrenia that has been notoriously difficult to treat. Many current antipsychotics primarily focus on dopaminergic systems, but they tend to leave cognitive and negative symptoms unaddressed. Cobenfy's mechanism, which is focused on enhancing the cholinergic activity in the central nervous system, could fill a critical gap by improving cognitive processing, attention, and other executive functions, all of which are crucial for patient quality of life.

As a result, the use of Cobenfy may prompt a shift in schizophrenia treatment paradigms, where medications are tailored to more effectively target the wide range of symptoms experienced by patients. This shift may lead to more holistic treatment approaches that involve not only managing psychosis but also improving cognition and social functioning. It may also encourage the development of new drugs aimed at more specific targets within the muscarinic receptor family, potentially paving the way for even more personalized treatments for schizophrenia and related disorders.

Ongoing Research and Development

Research into Cobenfy and similar therapies is ongoing, as scientists continue to explore the full potential of cholinergic systems in treating psychiatric disorders. As of now, Cobenfy has shown promise in clinical trials for schizophrenia, but the research community remains keen to further explore its efficacy, safety, and applicability in various patient populations.

One of the key areas of ongoing research is the potential for long-term use of Cobenfy. The current clinical studies have primarily focused on short-term (up to one year) safety and efficacy, but understanding its long-term effects is crucial. Researchers are studying how Cobenfy impacts patients over extended periods and whether its effects on cognition and other domains remain consistent or improve with prolonged use.

Another area of focus is combining Cobenfy with other therapies. Given the complex nature of schizophrenia, treatment regimens often require more than one approach. Cobenfy might eventually be studied in combination with traditional antipsychotics or cognitive-behavioral therapy (CBT) to see whether this multi-pronged approach can provide more comprehensive treatment, especially for those who experience treatment-resistant schizophrenia.

The research is also expanding into examining the drug's potential use in treating other neuropsychiatric disorders. Disorders such as Alzheimer's disease or Parkinson's disease dementia, where cognitive impairment is a significant issue, may benefit from the cholinergic effects of xanomeline. If future studies confirm its applicability in these areas, Cobenfy could have a broader impact beyond just schizophrenia, offering more options for individuals with other challenging neurodegenerative conditions.

Expanding Applications for Cobenfy

While Cobenfy was initially developed as a treatment for schizophrenia, its unique pharmacological profile could make it useful in a wider range of neuropsychiatric and neurological disorders. Researchers are investigating whether Cobenfy can address cognitive deficits associated with other psychiatric disorders, such as bipolar disorder or major depressive disorder, where patients often experience significant cognitive impairment in addition to mood disturbances.

In particular, the role of cholinergic systems in cognition and emotional regulation suggests that Cobenfy might be useful in treating cognitive dysfunction in diseases like Alzheimer's disease. Cholinergic dysfunction is known to play a role in the cognitive decline observed in Alzheimer's, and drugs that enhance cholinergic activity have shown promise in early-stage clinical trials for Alzheimer's patients. Although Cobenfy's primary focus is on schizophrenia, its potential application in Alzheimer's treatment could be explored further, especially as the demand for treatments targeting cognitive decline grows.

Another potential expansion for Cobenfy is in the management of Parkinson's disease dementia. Similar to Alzheimer's, Parkinson's disease often results in cognitive decline, and some studies have suggested that modulating cholinergic receptors can help improve cognitive performance. Cobenfy's unique mechanism might prove beneficial in improving cognition in Parkinson's patients who experience both motor symptoms and dementia, thereby offering a new treatment option in this challenging aspect of Parkinson's disease.

Finally, the versatility of Cobenfy might extend to other neurological disorders, particularly those associated with neurocognitive deficits. As research continues to expand on the full impact of cholinergic modulation in the brain, it is likely that new therapeutic indications for Cobenfy will emerge, offering hope for individuals with a variety of cognitive-related disorders.

In conclusion, while Cobenfy has shown promising results for treating schizophrenia, its potential in the broader neuropsychiatric field is vast. Ongoing research will continue to unlock new uses for this medication, possibly altering the landscape of cognitive dysfunction treatment across multiple conditions. The future of Cobenfy lies not only in its application for schizophrenia but in its broader impact on mental health and neurological care.

Frequently Asked Questions

Common Concerns About Cobenfy

As with any new medication, patients and caregivers often have questions or concerns about Cobenfy (xanomeline and trospium chloride), especially regarding its safety and effectiveness. One common concern is the potential side effects of the drug. While Cobenfy is generally well-tolerated, it can cause adverse reactions such as nausea, dizziness, constipation, and hypertension. It is important for patients to discuss any concerns about these side effects with their healthcare provider, especially if they have pre-existing conditions or are taking other medications.

Another concern relates to the drug's mechanism of action, as Cobenfy is the first of its kind to target M1 and M4 muscarinic receptors rather than D2 receptors, which are targeted by traditional antipsychotics. Some patients may be unfamiliar with how this novel approach works and whether it is effective in managing schizophrenia symptoms. Healthcare providers can help clarify that Cobenfy is designed to offer a new treatment option by focusing on a different pathway in the brain, which may reduce the risk of certain side effects seen with traditional medications.

Lastly, there may be concerns regarding the cost of Cobenfy and its accessibility. However, programs like Cobenfy Cares™ have been designed to help alleviate financial and insurance burdens. These programs can assist eligible patients in managing the cost of the medication and ensure they have access to treatment.

Guidance for Patients and Caregivers

For patients and caregivers, one of the first steps when starting treatment with Cobenfy is understanding the potential risks and benefits. Patients should be fully informed about the common side effects, which include nausea, constipation, and dizziness, and know how to monitor for any adverse reactions. It is essential to maintain open communication with healthcare providers about any symptoms or concerns that arise during treatment.

Caregivers should be proactive in helping patients adhere to their prescribed regimen. They can assist by reminding patients to take their medication as directed and ensuring they attend follow-up appointments with their healthcare provider. Additionally, caregivers should be aware of any potential side effects that may affect the patient's daily activities, such as dizziness or gastrointestinal discomfort, and help manage those symptoms when possible.

If patients experience any severe side effects such as difficulty breathing or swelling of the face and throat (a sign of angioedema), they should seek immediate medical attention. It's important to always report new or unusual symptoms to a healthcare provider promptly to ensure the treatment is proceeding safely and effectively.

Insights for Healthcare Professionals

Healthcare professionals are integral in managing the introduction of Cobenfy into schizophrenia treatment regimens. Since Cobenfy represents a novel approach to managing the condition, professionals should thoroughly evaluate each patient's medical history to identify any potential contraindications, such as renal or hepatic impairment, that could increase the risk of side effects. It is essential to regularly monitor patients for common adverse reactions, including gastrointestinal issues, dizziness, and hypertension.

For patients with special populations, such as those with pre-existing renal or hepatic conditions, dose adjustments or careful monitoring may be required to minimize risks. Healthcare professionals should also counsel patients about the potential central nervous system effects, such as dizziness or confusion, and advise them not to engage in activities like driving or operating heavy machinery until they understand how Cobenfy affects them.

In addition to pharmacological management, healthcare professionals should be prepared to address any concerns patients may have about the cost and accessibility of Cobenfy. The Cobenfy Cares™ program can provide important resources for patients, so healthcare providers should ensure their patients are aware of this option. Overall, healthcare professionals play a key role in ensuring the effective and safe use of Cobenfy, helping patients achieve better outcomes while minimizing risks associated with the medication.

By understanding these concerns and providing appropriate guidance, both patients and healthcare professionals can make informed decisions about the treatment process and improve the management of schizophrenia with Cobenfy.

Conclusion

The Role of Cobenfy in Transforming Schizophrenia Care

Cobenfy (xanomeline and trospium chloride) represents a significant advancement in the treatment of schizophrenia, offering a novel approach to managing this complex and debilitating condition. Schizophrenia is often difficult to treat due to its multifaceted symptoms, which include positive, negative, and cognitive symptoms. Traditional antipsychotic medications primarily target dopamine receptors, which have been linked to various side effects such as motor dysfunction, weight gain, and sedation. In contrast, Cobenfy offers a unique mechanism of action by targeting M1 and M4 muscarinic receptors, which are believed to play a role in regulating cognitive function and emotional processing in the brain.

By focusing on these muscarinic receptors, Cobenfy may reduce the incidence of some of the side effects commonly seen with other antipsychotics, such as movement disorders. The combination of xanomeline, a muscarinic receptor agonist, and trospium chloride, an agent that helps mitigate peripheral side effects, allows Cobenfy to provide therapeutic benefits without exacerbating certain issues associated with typical treatments. This breakthrough in treatment is especially important because schizophrenia remains one of the leading causes of disability worldwide, affecting millions of people, yet treatment options have been limited.

Cobenfy's clinical trials have shown promising results in reducing the symptoms of schizophrenia, demonstrating both efficacy and safety in managing the condition. In Phase 3 studies such as EMERGENT-2 and EMERGENT-3, Cobenfy significantly reduced symptoms as measured by the Positive and Negative Syndrome Scale (PANSS), a primary tool for evaluating schizophrenia severity. These findings have positioned Cobenfy as a potentially transformative option for patients who have not responded well to existing treatments or who experience intolerable side effects from them.

The Path Forward for Patients and Providers

As Cobenfy continues to gain recognition in the field of schizophrenia care, the path forward for patients and providers involves careful integration of this new treatment into clinical practice. For patients, the availability of Cobenfy represents a new opportunity for better management of their condition. However, it is essential for patients to work closely with their healthcare providers to assess whether Cobenfy is the right fit for their specific needs. This includes evaluating potential risks, especially in special populations such as those with renal or hepatic impairment, and monitoring for any side effects that may emerge during treatment.

The ongoing education of both patients and healthcare providers will be critical in optimizing the use of Cobenfy. For healthcare providers, understanding the unique mechanism of action of Cobenfy and how it differs from other antipsychotics will be essential in making informed treatment decisions. Providers should also stay informed about any new research and clinical findings related to Cobenfy, as ongoing studies may reveal additional benefits or considerations.

The role of patient support programs, such as Cobenfy Cares™, will also be vital in improving access to this medication for those who need it. These programs can help ease the financial burden that may accompany new treatments, ensuring that more patients have access to cutting-edge therapies like Cobenfy.

Looking ahead, there is great potential for further development in the treatment of schizophrenia. With medications like Cobenfy, we are moving towards a more nuanced approach to treating this complex condition. While there is still much to learn, particularly in terms of long-term safety and efficacy, Cobenfy's introduction has already marked an important step in transforming the landscape of schizophrenia care. As research and clinical experience continue to shape the future of treatment options, the ultimate goal remains clear: to improve the quality of life for individuals living with schizophrenia and help them achieve better mental health outcomes.

www.ingramcontent.com/pod-product-compliance
Lightning Source LLC
Chambersburg PA
CBHW082256220526
45469CB00009B/3025